We invite you tith
Chill & Spill,
book for co

Please note that stories submitted are subject to editorial approval and will be edited for length and grammar. The aim is to communicate capabilities and benefits of the program. Please submit your story to **chill@artwithheart.org** or write to us at the address below.

Proceeds from the sale of this book help **Art with Heart**, a nonprofit organization that empowers youth in crisis through creative books and programs that foster self-expression. Please consider donating today:

Art with Heart | P.O. Box 94402, Seattle, WA 98124-6702
info@artwithheart.org | www.artwithheart.org
phone: 206.362.4047 | fax: 206.277.7836

ISBN 0-9715240-7-6. **A Therapist's Companion to Chill & Spill**. Printed in the U.S. ©2006 Art with Heart. All rights reserved. First Printing: September 2006.

This book is intended to be used in tandem with Art with Heart's "Chill & Spill" journal. No part of this book may be used or reproduced in any manner or in any medium whatsoever without prior written permission from the Publisher.

DISCLAIMER: The authors and publisher of this book assume no responsibility or liability for direct, special or consequential damages or other damages of any kind whatsoever which, for any reason whatsoever, arise in connection with direct or indirect use. Chill and Spill can be an effective part of treatment, but should not the treatment plan in and of itself. Participation does not ensure in-school success, abstinence from drug use or refrainment from suicide or suicidal behaviors. The activities are not meant as a substitute for individualized mental health therapy provided in person by a professional. Art with Heart makes no claim, promise or guarantee to cure, treat, diagnose or otherwise provide mental or behavioral health.

TO ORDER THIS AND OTHER ART WITH HEART PUBLICATIONS, PLEASE VISIT
WWW.ARTWITHHEART.ORG/SHOP

ART WITH HEART
healing kids through creativity

Contents

Chill & Spill: The Need 4

The Intended Audience / Goals for Chill & Spill 5

Settings / Age-Appropriate Illustrations................................... 6

Various Approaches to Presentation.. 7

Working in Tandum with an Artist or Writer 7

What is Art Therapy? 8

Using Expressive Arts to Support Trauma Recovery.................... 9-10

Using Chill & Spill in a Group Setting 11

Frequently Asked Questions 12-15

Chill & Spill Page by Page 16

     Writing & Drawing Can Help 17

     The Best Three Words to Describe ME 18

     Your Place 19

     Fly Away... 20

     Exclusive Interview 21

     Me, Myself and I..22

     How Others See Me/See Myself/Want to be Seen (trifold).....23

     And I Really Do Feel 24

     Circle Journey, Mandala: Part 1 25

     Circle Journey, Mandala: Part 2................................ 26

     Inside of Me..27

     Lifeline (tri-fold) 28

     Powerful-Powerless 29

     Action I Reaction 30

     Dream Diary...31

     Shoulda Woulda Coulda 32-33

     The Last Word 34-35

     Bridges.. 36-37

Glossary..38-40

Stories from the Field 41-43

About Art with Heart.. 44

About the Authors.. 45

Ordering information 46

Ordering Form.. 47

Therapist's Survey 48-49

Chill & Spill: The Need

The Adverse Childhood Experiences (ACE) Study, a collaborative effort between the Centers for Disease Control and Prevention and Kaiser Permanente's Department of Preventative Medicine, revealed a powerful relationship between emotional childhood experiences and physical and mental health as adults. Early adverse experiences are vastly more common than recognized and have a powerful relation to mental and physical health even a half-century later.[1] According to the National Center for PTSD, children and adolescents who have experienced traumatic events often exhibit associated symptoms such as major depression, substance abuse, separation anxiety, panic disorder, generalized anxiety disorder, and externalizing disorders such as attention-deficit/hyperactivity disorder, oppositional defiant disorder and conduct disorder.[2]

Art therapists and other professionals working with troubled youth believe that by incorporating the creative process in treatment, clients are better able to communicate difficult issues, reduce stress and normalize feelings in ways that oftentimes can be too difficult during talk therapy. The process of art-making can be soothing and rewarding. Clients gain insight as they give expression to the inexpressible and creative decisions are illuminated through therapist's open-ended questions.

Chill & Spill is a unique and eclectic therapeutic tool to aid trauma recovery utilizing cognitive behavioral, narrative and art therapies. The book was designed to encourage emotional intelligence in a developmentally useful way, enlisting the user as an active participant in his or her own emotional recovery.

The **Therapist's Companion** was developed by a team of Mental Health Professionals in an effort to increase Chill & Spill's effectiveness in helping youth recover from traumatic experiences. Therapists and counselors who have not yet utilized the expressive arts in their practice will benefit by gaining knowledge of the concepts and therapies behind the activities found in Chill & Spill.

An **Artist's & Writer's Guide** is being developed and will also be available on www.artwithheart.org/shop for those who wish to create a cohesive Chill & Spill program.

---

1   http://www.acestudy.org
2   Http://www.ncptsd.va.gov/facts/specific/fs_children.html

The Intended Audience

Chill & Spill benefits adolescents and young adults suffering from various difficulties and issues such as:

- Anxiety / depression
- Grief / loss
- Low self esteem
- Personal/sexual identity
- Self-harm issues
- Eating disorders
- Substance abuse
- Trauma recovery
- School crisis
- Family / relationship issues
- Anger management
- Social development
- PTSD
- Serious or chronic illness
- Domestic violence
- Emotional/physical/sexual abuse

Goals for the Chill & Spill Program

The activities found in **Chill & Spill** are meant to promote:

- Self-acceptance
- Self-expression
- Self-awareness
- Self-realization
- Self-reliance
- Positive decision making
- Emotional intelligence
- Hope & inspiration
- Positive communication
- Problem solving skills
- Empathy-building
- Coping strategies

The process of art-making and creative expression can help youth make sense of their experiences and communicate grief and loss. It allows them to become active participants in their own healing, helping them see themselves as survivors rather than victims; a critical step in trauma recovery.

Chill & Spill's layout brings the client on a progressive journey. It begins with non-threatening, confidence-building activities and slowly leads them towards trauma exploration. The ending activities lead them back to safety through closure and aspiration. Five blank pages follow each printed page to allow room for creative expression. A secondary blank book may be utilized if more room is needed.

EACH YOUTH NEEDS TO RECEIVE THEIR OWN BOOK. The Chill & Spill program is effective because it gives clients a safe place for complete and total expression. An important component of the healing process is the ability to reference older drawings and entries to chart emotional progress.

Settings

Chill & Spill can be used in a variety of settings such as:

- Group / individual therapy
- Hospitals / clinics
- Foster care / home
- Wellness centers
- Shelters
- Summer camps
- Nature programs
- Classrooms / school
- Juvenile detention / courts
- Mentor relationships
- Private practice
- Youth development programs
- Residential treatment facilities

Age-Appropriate Illustrations

The therapies behind the activities are not apparent to the client. This was deliberate and implemented through the choice of illustrators, who were chosen for their unique ability to visually relate to this hard-to-reach population. Youth will recognize their artistic styles from television, music, magazines, products and books. **The non-clinical look makes the activities less threatening and helps clients enter the therapeutic process without hindrance.** The art is intended to inspire free-flowing, creative thought as well as to "give permission" to express themselves in whatever medium and form they are comfortable with.

The illustrations also serve a secondary use: ask your client to study the printed artwork as you go through the book together and encourage discussions about them.

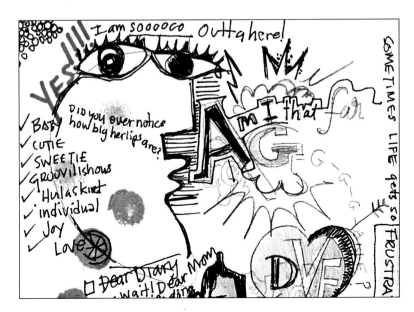

Various Approaches to Presentation

Therapists, School Counselors and Child Life Specialists each use Chill & Spill differently, depending on the needs of the teens they serve. You can use the book as:

- **An ice-breaker** to help begin a dialogue
- **Incentive** for program or therapy participation
- **Curriculum** for group or individual therapy
- **A mentorship outreach** tool that helps to guide the relationship
- **A youth peer outreach** tool allowing youth who have experienced the book to introduce it to others
- **Assertiveness training** to help teach confidence and expression skills
- **School curriculum or extra-curricular programming** such as a creative writing assignments, expressive art projects, journaling club, etc.
- **A non-threatening introduction** to journaling, poetry, songwriting or creative writing projects

Working in Tandem with an Artist or Writer

This Therapist's Companion was created to enhance your success in your work with Chill & Spill. It outlines ideas for creative expansion that are easy to do with limited artistic skills and supplies. We are also developing an **Artist's & Writer's Guide** to create a holistic program, allowing you to work in tandem with a professional artist or writer who can enrich the group experience and introduce other mediums and skills appropriate to healthy self-expression. At the end of the workshop, clients will likely have produced a piece of artwork or creative writing that can be used to facilitate discussion, opening the path for a more dynamic and integrated session that will be both participatory and fulfilling.

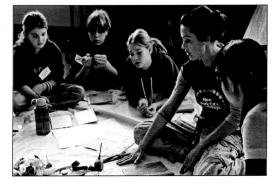

What is Art Therapy?

Art therapy was first practiced in England in the 1940s as a result of a collaboration between artist Adrian Hill and psychotherapist Irene Champernowne. Today, it is practiced throughout the world and is used to help people that suffer from emotional and psychological problems, as well as those who merely wish to discover more about themselves.

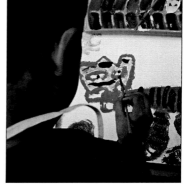

Art therapy integrates the fields of human development, visual art and the creative process with models of counseling and psychotherapy. It incorporates the creative process of art-making, such as drawing, painting or sculpture, in order to express one's feelings and release emotional tension.

Art therapy is used to assess and treat anxiety, depression and other mental and emotional problems and disorders; mental illness; substance abuse and other addictions; family and relationship issues; abuse and domestic violence; social and emotional difficulties related to disability and illness; trauma and loss; physical, cognitive and neurological problems; and psychosocial difficulties related to medical illness.

It can have a powerful healing effect on the client. Emotions that are too deep for words often find a way to surface. This form of therapy helps people overcome difficult feelings, develop interpersonal skills, manage behavior, increase self-esteem and self-awareness and ideally leads to greater physical well-being.

Art therapists are masters level professionals who hold a degree in art therapy or a related field. Educational requirements include: theories of art therapy, counseling and psychotherapy; ethics and standards of practice; assessment and evaluation; individual, group and family techniques; human and creative development; multicultural issues; research methods; and practicum experiences in clinical, community, and/or other settings. Art therapists are skilled in the application of a variety of art modalities for assessment and treatment.[3]

---

3 http://www.arttherapy.org

Using Expressive Arts to Support Trauma Recovery

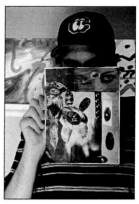

Art and writing are natural forms of communication for adolescents because it is often easier for them to express themselves visually than verbally. This is particularly true for those who have experienced a traumatic life event. The following guidelines may be helpful to you as you begin your use of the expressive arts through this Chill & Spill Companion:

- **Ease into the artistic activity** by allowing the clients to debrief or "check in" before beginning the session.

- **Make various materials available** such as pencils, colored pencils, oil pastels, markers, collage materials such as pre-cut magazine images, wrapping paper, old stamps, boxes, tissue paper, glue sticks or PVA glue, tape. **NOTE:** Collage is considered a "safe" medium for those who do not feel comfortable drawing since it is easy to control, provides structure and stimulates imagination.

- **Encourage clients to express themselves** in whatever creative way they are comfortable (doodling, drawing, poetry, songs, stories, abstract coloring). Remember that age, personality, ability, interest and skill level will influence both their choices and output.

- **Inform clients about transitions** to help ease them from one part of the activity to another by keeping them informed about the process. Stress related to unpredictability can be alleviated by making the workshop's time line clear (for example: "First we will work on finding collage images for 10 minutes and then we will start assembling what we've found."). Be sure to allow for flexibility within the schedule as appropriate.

- **Do not be tempted to draw or paint for them**, but be attentive and supportive, providing instruction if he or she does not know how to use a material, brush or tool. Respect their ability.

- **Focus on the experience and process** rather than the end product. Refrain from instructing the client on a "correct" way to visually communicate an idea and allow them to find their own way. It is not about creating "pretty" pictures or writing and re-writing to perfection.

- **Do not feel that you need to specifically address the trauma** in order for the session to be productive. Artistic activity can be productive and healthy in and of itself.

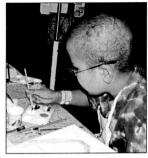

- **Let their art speak to you,** but don't assume you know why they chose to draw or collage particular images. Attention to the art that is produced gives the therapist some idea of the client's concerns and life circumstances. Engage in a dialogue by simply asking them to describe the elements in their picture or story. Encourage storytelling about what they've produced and accept what is communicated. Reserve personal projections about what you think the images mean and allow the client to reveal the metaphors behind their artwork. Establish a principle of neutrality from the beginning in order to gain greater trust. The most accurate assessment comes from comparing what is produced from session to session and noting variations that occur both in the content and the verbal explanations of its meaning.

- **Allow the client to use artistic expression** in a variety of ways. Some clients will repeat images of the traumatic event in their journal while others may resist memories of the actual event, preferring to use art activities to soothe and reduce stress. Both ways are acceptable.

- **Offer a closing activity** to reassure them such as tidying up or deep breathing. It is important that the client feels calm and in control as significant and personal feelings may have been exposed that may cause them to feel at-risk for rejection.

- **Offer discussion questions** (see the "Chill & Spill Page by Page" section for salient discussion points) to help them understand what the process revealed to them.

- **Allow for the possibility** that the client will not share the finished product with you. Praise the fact that they've communicated a boundary to you and respect their desire to keep certain things private. This can be especially important for children who have suffered physical and sexual abuse.[4]

---

4 Healing Arts for Tsunami Survivors: Using Art Activities to Support Trauma Recovery in Children, a joint publication of the International Children's Art Foundation (www.icaf.org) and the American Art Therapy Association, Inc., January 2005.

Using Chill & Spill in a Group Setting

Chill & Spill can be used for self-guided discovery, but we recommend it be used within the context of a therapeutic relationship, where it can be adapted for individual or group therapy. Groups are an effective way to utilize limited resources when time constraints cause challenges. The ideas below will help you create an effective group experience:

- In **Time-Limited Groups**, use Chill & Spill as curriculum to provide structure, implementing one page per session. Depending on how often your group meets, target activities that are the most salient, introducing the book in the first session to give them a working knowledge of it. Instruct the group to use the first half of the session to work silently and individually on the chosen activity and then open up discussion about what they discovered about themselves during their time.

- Because members have varying backgrounds and issues in **Heterogeneous Groups**, the therapist can assign pages as homework, asking clients to bring the completed task to the next session to share what was revealed to them. Even if a client does not complete the assignment, they will benefit from hearing what the others share. They can be asked to articulate what they learned from listening to the other participants.

- Adapt the activity pages for **Single-Issue or Skill-Development Groups** to focus on a related problem area (for example: a school crisis victims group can focus on the grief and loss pages, an anger management group can focus on the trigger activities and an eating disorder group can focus on body image activities). Empower the group by asking them to choose an issue they need to work on. Then have them review the book, choosing particular pages that relate to that topic to focus upcoming sessions on. Allow flexibility to spend more time on a particular page as needed, even extending a particular activity over a series of weeks, so as not to force the pace.

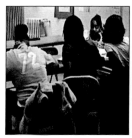
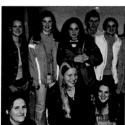
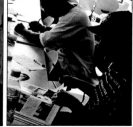

Frequently Asked Questions

WHAT'S SPECIAL ABOUT THE THERAPIES IN CHILL & SPILL? Cognitive behavioral, narrative and art therapies lie hidden beneath layers of eye-catching and age-appropriate artwork. The therapies behind Chill & Spill can help reduce symptoms of distress and build skills that improve youth's abilities to handle future stress and trauma. Symptom reduction is accomplished by reducing maladaptive thinking and anxiety directly through creative expression. The psyche is revealed not only through words, but through images, colors, symbols and metaphors. It helps clients process traumatic experiences, reducing grief and increasing emotional intelligence. The interplay of writing and drawing allows them to "let go", express and release as well as gain insight by studying metaphoric messages that appear.

CAN CHILL & SPILL BE USED IN PREVENTION OR EARLY INTERVENTION? Absolutely. The primary reasons for intervening early with an at-risk teen are to provide support and assistance to maximize positive growth and head-off potentially unhealthy behaviors such as substance abuse. Early intervention can result in the teen experiencing fewer school or relational problems and needing fewer rehabilitation services later in life.

THE TEENS I SERVE HAVE SOME SERIOUS PROBLEMS. HOW WILL CHILL & SPILL HELP? Traumatic life events can lead to impairment (including behavioral problems and functional impairment), and these in turn can lead to long-term adjustment problems such as PTSD, depression, violent behavior and substance abuse. These adverse outcomes, in turn, increase risk for exposure to more traumatic events and life stressors, compounding vulnerability in the future, creating a cycle of maladaptive behavior. Chill & Spill is especially helpful for those who cannot or will not express themselves verbally. Drawing and writing help youth process difficult emotions and can illuminate solutions.

WHAT'S THE BEST WAY TO APPROACH TEENS WITH THIS BOOK? We have seen great success when the book is used as incentive for participation, as something youth earn through compliance, as homework assignments or as curriculum for group therapy.

CAN I WORK THROUGH THE BOOK WITH THE TEEN? That depends on the teen. If you have established an open and trusting relationship, you may be able to. It is best to leave your direct level of involvement up to the teen.

THEY WON'T SHARE THEIR BOOK WITH ME. CAN I SNEAK A PEEK?
No. Do not betray their trust. Chill & Spill is a private journal that helps them express their innermost thoughts and fears; allow it to be as sacred as a diary. If they feel you might look, they will write with you in mind, defeating the purpose. You can encourage them to share, but accept the boundaries they create.

WHAT IF I DON'T KNOW WHAT TO SAY WHEN THEY DO SHARE THEIR DRAWINGS WITH ME? Keep your comments and questions open-ended, saying things such as: Tell me about your picture. Tell me about the colors you chose. What does this drawing make you feel like? Why did you choose that image? What does this image mean to you?

WHAT DO I SAY TO THE TEEN WHO SAYS THEY CAN'T OR DON'T WANT TO DRAW? Oftentimes, resistance stems from lack of confidence or fear of failure. When people say, "I can't draw", what they mean is "I can't draw what I see in my head." Artistic ability actually does not matter. Encourage the client by saying, "If you can draw a stick man or scribble, you can do this because it's the meaning behind the drawing that really matters and what you discover about yourself while you do the activities." Each person gains self-awareness and insight from the images that come from the unconscious mind and become clues to challenges, behaviors and feelings. Help them risk being "wrong," help them to be willing to put something down without censoring it. By praising their efforts in a non-judgemental way and providing positive feedback, you will help them gain confidence in their own ability.

I LIKE THE IDEA OF DOING COLLAGE. ARE THERE ANY THINGS I SHOULD BE AWARE OF? Collage is an outstanding activity for clients of any artistic ability. Challenge them not to use "ready-made images" (such as a model's face) but to create their own new images by finding various parts from different pages to create a unique face (lips from one page, eyebrows cut out from an image of hair, clothes from patterns and backgrounds) that will metaphorically reflect their unique feelings. For teens who have body or self-esteem issues, we recommend that you choose magazines that don't dwell on the fashions or celebrities.

I HAVE A GROUP OF KIDS WHO ARE "HUFFERS." WHAT ART SUPPLIES SHOULD I AVOID? If you work with youth who deliberately inhale fumes to produce mood-altering effects, look for art supplies marked "non-toxic" such as Elmer's Glue, Modge Podge or glue sticks, colored pencils or water-based acrylic paint. For other

A Therapist's Companion to Chill & Spill | page 13

ideas, see the "Acceptable Children's Art and Craft Materials" list of 2,500 non-toxic art materials available from the California Department of Health Services. Avoid rubber cement, printing inks, spray paints, correction fluid, certain permanent, "magic" and other solvent-based markers including Sharpies.[5]

WHAT IF THE BOOK BRINGS UP THINGS I'M NOT COMFORTABLE DISCUSSING? If traumatic stories are shared and something is revealed that distresses you, remain calm. Do not act with alarm in front of the client. Encourage them to express their feelings, even if you don't agree or it's painful to hear. Lecturing or advice-giving may cause them to withdraw further.

For teens that have faced a traumatic experience, you can help in the following ways:[6]

- Encourage them to talk about their feelings and tell their story.

- Do not force expression of the traumatic event, but let them know that it is normal to feel upset, angry, or afraid when something bad happens.

- Create a safe place for expression and communication, free from judgment and criticism. Listen and respond without judgment or interpretation; be open and encouraging.

- Be open to ongoing conversations.

- Be sure to understand and manage your own feelings about the traumatic event. Take time to prepare yourself emotionally before you attempt to reassure your teen.

- Help them feel safe by asking them about their specific needs for comfort.

- Listen actively, asking open-ended questions. When appro-priate, re-frame what you think you heard and "play it back" to make sure you understood what they were trying to say.

- Provide structure and routine whenever possible while being flexible to their needs; allow them to make some decisions about routines and other aspects of daily life if possible.

- Be aware that memories and feelings about these losses are recurrent and can be triggered by everyday images and reminders of the person or event.

---

5 Spandorfer M, Curtiss D, Snyder J. Making Art Safely. New York: Van Nostrand Reinhold, 1993
6 Ibid

- It is particularly important that you normalize any feelings expressed by letting them know that others have experienced the same emotions. Help them feel connected to peers and adults who can provide support and decrease isolation.
- Realize that teens that are experiencing loss will need additional support for an extended period of time.
- Recognize your competency level and limitations. The issue may be beyond your training and what you are able to responsibly handle. If you have a therapeutic alliance (relationship of trust) with the client, refer them to another professional who has more knowledge in the matter.

WHAT KIND OF RESULTS CAN I EXPECT? Each individual is unique and expresses himself or herself differently. The goal of Chill & Spill is to help the client grow to understand their own feelings better, become able to express feelings appropriately, feel more secure and have a healthier self-esteem. The book has the potential of helping teens increase emotional awareness by discovering their own patterns and triggers. The activities can help them develop strategies to change negative behavior. Thoughts and emotions naturally become more accessible during the act of creative expression. Through the use of the book, we hope you will be able to deepen and enrich your practice through the expressive arts.

WHO HAS CHILL & SPILL HELPED SO FAR? Shortly after Chill & Spill was first printed, Hurricane Katrina created havoc for thousands of children and their families in the gulf states. Art with Heart was able to provide books to thousands of high school students affected by the disaster. Since then, Chill & Spill has been successfully used in residential treatment centers, in middle and high schools, by homeless shelters and hospitals across North America. **We welcome hearing how Chill & Spill helped you reach kids as well.** Write to us at Art with Heart, P.O. Box 94402, Seattle, WA 98124-6702.

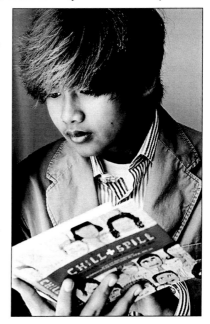

Chill & Spill Page by Page

Chill & Spill is most effective if you have an awareness of the concepts and therapeutic goals behind each activity. We have included "Ideas for Variation" to help you expand the activities in both a group or individual basis, along with supportive questions and discussion points that will help you elicit responses and create a healthy dialog with your clients.

We created Chill & Spill with a deliberate "flow," moving the client from trust-building activities to closure-building activities. We recommend that you follow the book in its given order and that **each youth receive their own book** to give them a place they will feel free to express their true, innermost feelings. The following pages will help you create an experience that meets your client's particular needs and assists them on their healing journey.

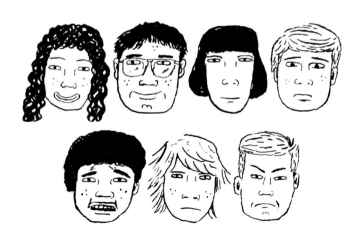

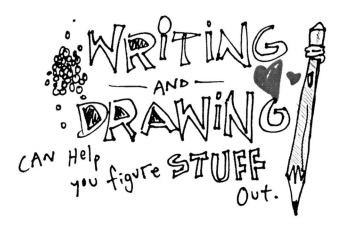

ACTIVITY GOALS

This activity allows the client to take ownership of the book and engage in relationship-building with the therapist. It promotes free-flowing thought and feeling, initiates conversation and helps establish trust.

IDEAS FOR VARIATION

- Ask the client to take the activity one step further and use the pages to explore feelings, thoughts and goals or ask them to use these pages daily over the next week, summarizing things that affect them.

- Encourage the client to experiment with color, asking them to choose color markers or pencils that represent different moods, creating their own color code system. Ask them to note any patterns.

- Use as a free-association group activity, using prompts to help them begin ("Yesterday after lunch, I felt…", "The most important thing is…").

OPTIONAL MATERIALS

Waterproof colored markers; colored pencils, pencil sharpener

DISCUSSION POINTS

- **Q:** Why is finding a way to express emotions important?
- **Q:** How can journaling, drawing or doodling be beneficial?
- Discuss the huge variety of emotions and introduce the concept of "emotional intelligence."

The Best Three Words to Describe Me

ACTIVITY GOALS
This activity creates ownership and trust of the book/the process. It helps build the client's identity, raises self-esteem and encourages goal setting. It allows the therapist to join them in exploring what's important to the client and what their artwork and/or writing means. It also helps the facilitator establish a rapport with the client and leads to better communication.

IDEAS FOR VARIATION
- Ask them to use what they've written in the book to form a personal symbol/logo that represents who they are. Encourage them to use it throughout the book and sign their pages with it.
- Ask the client create a story about their heroes, skills, life, goals, etc. based on what they wrote for this page.
- Have the client write a Top Ten list of things they are good at or things they want to accomplish over the next ten years.
- Ask them use some of the illustrations found along the border to create a rebus story introducing themselves to a new person.
- Create a visual "short story" of their life – either in the journal, or on cards for each "chapter" – using the illustrations on the page as prompts.

OPTIONAL MATERIALS
3x5 cards, waterproof markers; colored pencils, pencil sharpener

DISCUSSION POINTS
- **Q:** Was it easy or hard to come up with the descriptive words?
- **Q:** Are the words you chose helpful or hurtful? Do they reflect the way you see yourself or the way you think others see you?
- **Q:** Was it easy or hard to write about things you are good at?
- Ask them to share (if they are comfortable doing so) important moments in their personal short story.

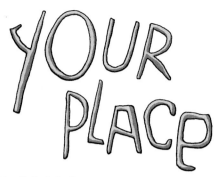

YOUR PLACE

ACTIVITY GOALS

This activity helps establish a real or imaginary "safe place" for clients to revisit when difficulties arise. It encourages clients to access the power of their imaginations through creation or identification of a peaceful, playful or healing space. This is a tool-building activity that encourages self-awareness.

IDEAS FOR VARIATION

- Take the clients through a guided imagery to help them find a safe place where they cannot be hurt.
- Ask them to draw a map of the area surrounding their safe place (similar to a treasure map). Ask them to talk about their journey to get there: what they feel, experience along the way.
- Ask them to create an inventory of items that are found in their safe place and write about why those items are special.

OPTIONAL MATERIALS

Waterproof color markers, shoe boxes, cardboard, scissors, glue sticks or PVA glue, found objects, magazines

DISCUSSION POINTS

- **Q:** Do you have a safe place? Why does it make you feel safe? What makes it different from other places?
- **Q:** How do you enter and exit out of your safe place?
- **Q:** What are the benefits of having a safe place? When can you use it?
- Discuss why self-care is important and talk about progressive relaxation techniques.

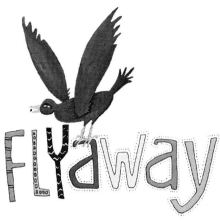

ACTIVITY GOALS

This activity is another way to establish a "safe place." It also allows reflective distance by exploring the association between nature and feelings. It is a strength-building activity and helps them access their imagination, creativity and story-telling skills.

IDEAS FOR VARIATION

- Ask the client to identify their support group, asking what roles each person would take in their growth and nurturing. Have them write short poem about their growth.
- Provide actual seeds, soil and a pot. Have them decorate the pots with words or images that are edifying and nurturing. This activity helps them build empathy, nurturing and ownership. Talk to them about what happens if the seed doesn't get enough (or gets too much) water or sun.

OPTIONAL MATERIALS

Easy to grow seeds (nasturtium, radish, beans), small container with drainage hole, bagged sterile potting soil, waterproof color markers, acrylic paint, brushes, water containers, newspaper to protect the furniture

DISCUSSION POINTS

- **Q:** How do you take care of yourself? Do you make time to do that?
- Discuss any themes that present themselves in their artwork or writings and explore the deeper meanings.
- Discuss their support structure and feelings of safety and comfort.
- Help them practice esteem-building by verbalizing personal needs.

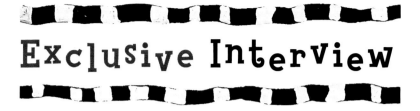

Exclusive Interview

ACTIVITY GOALS

This activity builds identity and self-esteem. It allows free expression within a structured and safe environment. The healthy fantasy helps them manifest their desired reality. Further exploration of this activity can help build confidence in communicating desires and can increase interpersonal, social and assertiveness skills.

IDEAS FOR VARIATION

- Add specific interview questions that are relevant to the clients.
- Ask them to create a collage based on one of the questions.
- Expand the interview to include their career possibilities or, as homework, ask them to interview those in their support structure.
- Have clients interview each other and take photos of each other.
- Read them interviews of folks who have experienced difficult childhoods who are now successful, pointing out what might have affected their outcome (examples: Oprah, Dr. Wayne Dyer, Mary J. Blige, Eddie Murphy, Maya Angelo, Malcolm X, Dave Thomas of Wendy's).

OPTIONAL MATERIALS

Digital or Polaroid camera with film, biographies from the library

DISCUSSION POINTS

- **Q:** What can you do to make a difference in the world? In your neighborhood? Do you have the power to do that? Why or why not?
- **Q:** How comfortable are you in approaching people and successfully taking risks? How do you talk to people you don't know very well?
- Discuss how they see themselves in relation to others?
- Discuss the benefits and difference between dependence, independence and interdependence.

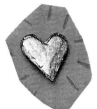

Me, Myself and I

ACTIVITY GOALS
This activity asks clients to identify images that represent themselves, allowing them to highlight their unique feelings, experiences and perspectives. It encourages them to value and explore their identity.

IDEAS FOR VARIATION
- Have the clients collage to illustrate two main ideas: 1. What Others Want Me To Be/Look Like and 2. Who I Really Am, to help them explore their concept of body image and confidence.

- Do a full-size body tracing (or trace their hand or face if there is limited space) on butcher paper. Cut out the tracing and give them a secondary theme that have not explored yet (a feeling, recent event, goal, memory, self-image, etc.) to collage or draw.

- Create a "family crest" (could also be their support group or family of choice) that represents personal identity, cultural heritage, ethnicity and supportive relationships.

OPTIONAL MATERIALS
Glue sticks or PVA glue, magazines, scissors; butcher paper, pencils, waterproof colored markers

DISCUSSION POINTS
- **Q:** What symbols represent you? Why? What other symbols or themes show up in your collage that represent what you like, your history, goals or priorities?

- **Q:** How do you place yourself in relationship to your actual or chosen family? Discuss identification.

- If leading the family crest activity, ask how they feel they "fit" into the world and how cultural heritage, ethnicity, supportive relationships and personal identity (including sexual identity) help shape their opinion of themselves.

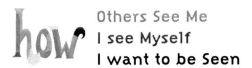

how Others See Me / I see Myself / I want to be Seen

ACTIVITY GOALS
This activity increases self-awareness, provides reflective distance, helps identify cognitive distortions and traps that block positive connection to others. **NOTE:** The inside of the tri-fold pages was designed specifically to provide privacy.

IDEAS FOR VARIATION
- Give each client a large piece of paper and ask them to draw, write or paint the attributes of "Who I am Today" on one side and "Who I Want to be Tomorrow" on the other side.
- Give each client a box, asking them to collage images of what their life would be like if they were at their highest potential on the outside. For the inside, have them collage or place objects and letters that represent private challenges they feel they have to overcome to reach their full potential.

OPTIONAL MATERIALS
Large paper or poster board; shoebox, glue sticks, magazines, scissors, acrylic paint, brushes, water containers

DISCUSSION POINTS
- **Q:** Do you feel that you have to have a specific image to be accepted? Discuss media, peer and other outside pressures.
- **Q:** Why is there a difference between the images? How does self-talk influence how your opinion of yourself and how others see you? How does this affect your ability, confidence, experiences?
- **Q:** What do you decide to keep private and what do you share with others? What's the difference between the two? What might happen if the "inside stuff" became "outside stuff?"
- **Q:** How do you keep your feelings safe? Discuss showing "faults," healthy boundaries and vulnerability.
- **Q:** How do you determine who to trust? Do you trust yourself?
- Explore the theme of societal and peer pressures.
- Discuss true self versus fase self.

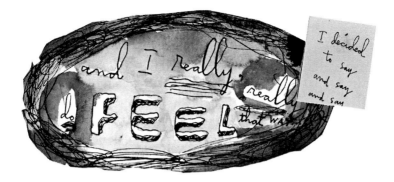

ACTIVITY GOALS

This activity creates structure while unlocking undiscovered feelings, desires and dreams. It uses free association to encourage unconscious insights which leads to increased self-awareness.

IDEAS FOR VARIATION

- Lead the activity by calling out the prompts, allowing 3-5 minutes in between each one.
- Ask clients to share one sentence from what they wrote that has personal meaning and discuss as a group.
- Ask the client to randomly circle three words that "stick out" to them and use them in a poem.
- Create a mask depicting a concept that one of the prompts brought up to encourage deeper self-expression and emotional awareness. Clients can use the mask to act out a scene or just "hide" behind it as they discuss difficult emotions.

OPTIONAL MATERIALS

Cardboard for mask base, oil pastels or acrylic paint, brushes, water containers, scissors, PVA glue, hole punch, rubber bands or elastic, collage materials such as yarn, felt, beads, feathers, etc.

DISCUSSION POINTS

- **Q**: How do you normally get your feelings out? How does it make you feel? Better or worse? How does this affect others?
- **Q**: Are there feelings that you can have and not share? Is it okay to keep some of your feelings private?
- Discuss the expression of feelings within a safe relationship.
- Explore how to expand emotional vocabulary.

CIRCLE JOURNEY
Mandala: Part 1

ACTIVITY GOALS

This activity guides the client through a relaxing journey of self-discovery through the application and exploration of color, lines, shapes and symbols. The nature theme in the Mandala encourages the client to think about the change, rebirth and renewal process. This may encourage reflection of the natural cycles in their lives.

IDEAS FOR VARIATION

- Guide the client to create a Mandala focused on a particular theme (their journey towards healing, redemption, forgiveness, gratefulness), choosing colors to represent moods and feelings.

- Create an abstract mosaic Mandala using unconventional materials such as beads, emphasizing mood, shape or color

- Cut out a big circle, dividing it into a "pie" with a slice for each group member. Ask each client to completely cover their slice with images of things that are personally representational in paint or collage. Each client should work individually and quietly, then bring the circle back together when finished.

OPTIONAL MATERIALS

Cardboard base, PVA glue and brush, yarn, beads, buttons, dried pasta and beans or small cut-out pieces from wrapping paper; scissors or box cutter, poster board, magazines, glue, acrylic paint, brushes, water container

DISCUSSION POINTS

- **Q:** How do you create balance in the different parts of your life between work, school, friends, family, fun, etc.? Are there any imbalances that you can see?

- If leading the "pie" activity above, ask: How did your perception change when you saw your piece as part of the whole? Discuss how each brings their own personality to the group and how the group fits together as a whole.

- Discuss how this activity can transfer to the activity on the following page (part 2) or to the creation of their own Mandalas whenever they need a relaxing activity.

A Therapist's Companion to Chill & Spill | page 25

CIRCLE JOURNEY
Mandala: Part 2

ACTIVITY GOALS

This activity helps clients identify and work through fear of change and overcome blocks by increasing their self-awareness and self-acceptance. It helps them see how fear impacts their lives and where imbalances might be. It empowers them to correct negative patterns and contain threatening feelings.

IDEAS FOR VARIATION

- On a separate piece of paper, have the client list out the fears they drew in the inner circle, along with an explanation. Help them work through any cognitive distortions of the fears by expanding on the ways those fears affect their lives.

- Pass out a separate sheet of paper that has a circle drawn on it that has been divided into 4 parts. Have them start from the middle point to create a secondary Mandala that represents balance, wholeness and healing.

- Ask the clients to translate the "strength" theme of their mandala into a collage, paying attention to image choices.

OPTIONAL MATERIALS

Print out of a circle divided into 4 parts, color markers, scissors, old magazines, glue stick

DISCUSSION POINTS

- **Q:** How can you change the negative messages and behavioral patterns that you've taken on because of you fears?

- **Q:** How does self-talk effect your daily life and decisions?

- Introduce the concept of physical and emotional triggers and what they look and/or feel like.

- Talk about positive versus maladaptive ways of coping.

- If relevant to the target group, provide education about the role of fear, discussing both the usefulness and potential destructiveness of fear. Model fact-checking to determine if fears are reasonable or unreasonable.

- Discuss how repeated practice can help them deal with fear.

A Therapist's Companion to Chill & Spill | page 26

iNsIde ★ oF me

ACTIVITY GOALS

This activity increases awareness, builds both a feeling and thought vocabulary and helps strengthen problem-solving skills.

IDEAS FOR VARIATION

- Have the client create a "Multi-Flow Map" pinpointing a time when they felt an overwhelming thought or emotion. Have them draw a rectangle (approximately 2x3 inches) in the center of the page and write a short phrase that summarizes that moment. On the left side of the rectangle, list the causes and on the right side, show the effects or consequences that happened as a result.

- Place a lamp on a table about 6 feet from a blank wall. Have the client stand against the wall so their profile casts a shadow. Tape a piece of paper to the wall and trace their silhouette. When the tracing is complete, ask them to color, draw or write their thoughts inside the face, asking them to show how much space each thought occupies.

OPTIONAL MATERIALS

Extra paper; desk lamp, large sheets of colored paper, tape, color markers or oil pastels

DISCUSSION POINTS

- **Q:** What happens when you let either your thoughts or your emotions lead? What happens when your thoughts and feelings don't agree? What do you do then?

- **Q:** Are there certain thoughts that take up a large portion of your time? When did that start? Is it connected to a certain event?

- Discuss patterns of thoughts and emotions (people, places or themes) that elicit overwhelming emotion. Discuss how to gain control over inappropriate repetitive thoughts.

personal lifeline

ACTIVITY GOALS

This activity creates pattern recognition and perspective through the process of honoring and exploring life events. It helps youth broaden their vantage point to ease anxiety, as well as increase value and empathy for their own unique life experiences.

IDEAS FOR VARIATION

- Have the client choose colors that represent happy, glad, sad and mad. Have them highlight each event in the representative color to show feelings associated with each event. Notice any patterns that become evident.

- On a second piece of paper, have them draw a graph showing more detail about life events in chronological order, mapping out things that affected them positively above the median and events that effected them negatively below the median.

- Have them create an imaginary lifeline starting tomorrow and ending in 10 years. Encourage them to draw pictures in place of words, using color to help associate feelings with new events.

OPTIONAL MATERIALS

Four different colors of highlighters per person; color markers, graph paper

DISCUSSION POINTS

- **Q:** Do you see any patterns, feelings, situations that seem to appear time and time again? Do they have anything to do with certain people, places or things or do they seem random?

- **Q:** Are there long periods of time that you remember being happy, glad, sad or mad? Are they connected with things on your lifeline?

- **Q:** How do you cope when both good and bad things happen?

- **Q:** What have you learned from things that have happened to you? How do you overcome difficult circumstances? How does what you've learned from the past change future decisions?

- Discuss life events that imprinted them negatively.

A Therapist's Companion to Chill & Spill I page 28

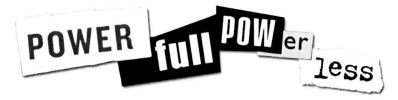

ACTIVITY GOALS
This activity assists youth in developing their own personal symbology, increasing self-awareness and allowing them to see themselves as valuable, capable and powerful.

IDEAS FOR VARIATION
- Choose other relationship words that are significant to the clients to illustrate (for example: victor/victim, freedom/addiction, love/hate).
- Ask the client to write several scenes of a play or a poem based on their artwork, which can then be acted out or red aloud. Have them create a cover for their creation, decorating it and giving it a title.
- Have the group play with the idea of extremes, discussing or acting out different scenes that illustrate relationship concepts. It is the group's responsibility to resolve each act, ending at a point of balance.

OPTIONAL MATERIALS
Extra paper for their play or poem, cardboard cover, string for binding book, color pencils, pencil sharpener

DISCUSSION POINTS
- **Q:** What about these images demonstrates powerful/powerless?
- **Q:** When in your life when you felt the most powerful? The most powerless?
- **Q:** What healthy ways can you use feelings of powerfulness and powerlessness? What are unhealthy ways to use these feelings?
- Pay attention to symbols that present themselves and ask open-ended questions, letting the client lead the discussion about the metaphors/meaning behind the images they chose.
- Explore the topic of duality of feeling: two vastly different emotions in the same person. Discuss the importance of maintaining balance.

Action | Reaction

ACTIVITY GOALS

This exercise helps clients clearly identify "hot buttons" or triggers they experience as a result of situations that cause them to feel reactive or emotionally/behaviorally out of control. By increasing awareness of physical and emotional clues, the client can learn and practice emotional regulation and coping skills to eliminate self-defeating thoughts and maladaptive behaviors.

IDEAS FOR VARIATION

- Ask them explore a particularly troubling trigger from their chart by detailing further ways they react that are harmful to themselves or harmful to others as well as alternative, healthy choices. Help them explore other coping strategies and bring them through a guided imagery that will help them role-play new ways of reacting.

- In a larger group, have participants act out to show their normal physical and emotional reactions to triggers. Have the group suggest alternative ways of responding and act out a corrective experience.

- Have the client create a pros and cons chart for their coping skills, having them label each as healthy or unhealthy. Explore what of their behavior "works" for them, what they gain or lose by acting that way, and what they would gain or lose by giving it up.

DISCUSSION POINTS

- **Q:** When this situation happens again, what choices are you going to make? How do you move from victim to victor?

- **Q:** If you can't change your circumstance, what can you change? Can you rise above it? Do you have a choice?

- Discuss decision-making, impulsive behavior, consequences and the relationship between them (cause/effect, action/reaction, empowerment/dis-empowerment).

- Discuss being empowered by their choices versus being a victim of their reactions; talk about real power versus false power.

- Discuss the victim/abuse cycle.

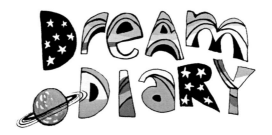

ACTIVITY GOALS

This activity can be extended over several weeks and will help clients become aware of both conscious and unconscious feelings. It encourages problem solving, self-awareness, self-discovery, pattern recognition and emotional intelligence. It can help them overcome fears and emotional dilemmas.

IDEAS FOR VARIATION

- Have client start their dream diary in **Chill & Spill** and continue in a blank notebook, kept by their bedside. Let them know that even dream fragments or feelings upon waking should be recorded. After a few weeks, ask them to notice re-occurring dreams and patterns. Empower them to self-interpret.

- Give each client a pillowcase, asking them to draw a picture of their favorite dream using fabric markers.

- Cut out stars and write down words on them that remind them of their favorite dreams, goals or wishes. Tape them on their ceiling (or in your office) to remind them of their aspirations.

OPTIONAL MATERIALS

Cotton pillowcases, fabric markers or fabric paint and brushes, cardboard to fit inside the case to prevent bleeding; markers, colored paper, scissors

DISCUSSION POINTS

- **Q:** What do your dreams mean to you? What symbols, people or themes have you noticed show up more than once? What do your dreams tell you about what you are going through right now?

- Encourage client to explore what their dreams are trying to tell them. Discuss the idea that everything the dreamer dreams is about the dreamer. From this perspective, what can be learned?

- Discuss the difference between "process" and "message" dreams.

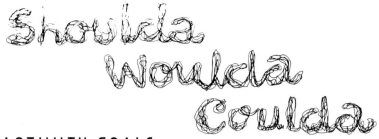

ACTIVITY GOALS:

This activity helps clients identify and externalize negative thoughts that block positive interactions with self and others (the Inner Critic). Through this awareness, they will learn to judge and discern the difference between messaging that is helpful or hurtful.

IDEAS FOR VARIATION

- In a loose and relaxed state, ask the client to use their non-dominant hand to draw or write negative messages they hear from their Inner Critic. Have them switch hands and write positive responses and messages with their dominant hand.

- Have the client write questions to themselves using their dominant hand and then switch and answer with their non-dominant hand.

- On a chalkboard or dry-erase board, have clients write or draw images of their negative self-talk. Then ask them to erase and "re-record" the message with words from a wiser perspective.

- Ask them to choose the message that is most troubling to them and, using the cartoon character they created in the initial activity, create a comic strip using humor to gain power.

- Ask them to keep a daily log, recording the messages they hear from their inner critic as they occur, noting details such as time of day, who was present, where they were, etc. Make note of patterns that begin to emerge.

- Have them write a "pink slip" (letter of dismissal) to the Inner Critic, remembering to thank them for their past help. Then have them write a new job description which will better serve their current needs and interests.

OPTIONAL MATERIALS

Dry-erase board and markers, eraser; color waterproof markers

DISCUSSION POINTS

- **Q:** What happens when we listen to the Inner Critic?
- **Q:** What does our Inner Critic keep us from doing that we want to do? What do we lose/gain from listening to it?
- **Q:** What's good about fear and when does fear hold us back? Discuss the function of fear.
- Discuss self-sabotage and how it keeps us from personal power.
- Discuss discernment between positive and negative messages.
- Discuss how the Inner Critic came to life as well as "survival value."

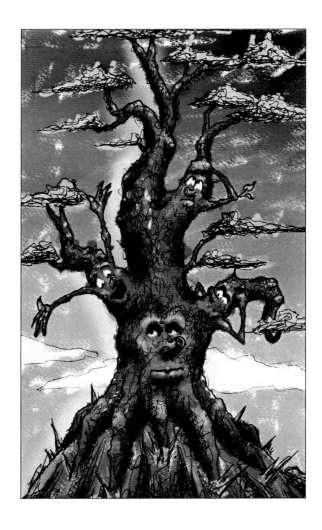

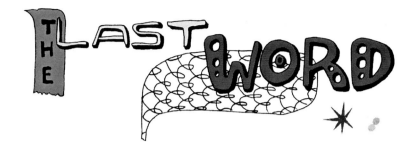

ACTIVITY GOALS
This activity gives closure and encourages healthy communication. Through reevaluation and normalization, the client is empowered as they process their grief or loss and gain greater context. By letting go, they allow space for new experiences.

IDEAS FOR VARIATION
- Have them switch roles (they are now the person they wrote to) and write a letter to themselves from that person's perspective.

- Have the client think of another "ghost" they need to let go of and forgive from their past and write a secondary letter to that person or event.

- Using the letter template as a guide, have each individual privately identify something they want to let go of (habit, behavior, relationship, goal or something they've outgrown) and write a letter to it. Have them go to the center of the group circle and verbally share a synopsis of what they are releasing. Have them dispose of their letter in a manner appropriate to their feelings. Sharing helps normalize their experience and deepens their learning from each other.

- Create a symbol or drawing of their loss out of natural objects (chalk on a rock, draw in the sand, twigs and twine, paint on paper, bread crumbs, etc.). Bring the objects outside to a quiet spot and give them time to reflect on the gifts they received from this loss before releasing it and leaving it behind in the elements. In a week, go back and visit the spot to see how nature renewed things. Note how nature breaks it down and allows it to become reabsorbed.

OPTIONAL MATERIALS
Trash can; chalk and rocks, twigs and twine, water soluble color markers and paper, or other natural materials

DISCUSSION POINTS

- **Q:** Why is it important that we acknowledge loss? What happens when we don't?

- **Q:** What did you gain from this loss? Why did you keep it with you for so long? How did it strengthen you? What lessons did you learn from it?

- **Q:** Why is gratefulness important? Why should we acknowledge that gift before we release it? How does being thankful affect your of peace of mind? Discuss gratitude's role.

- It is sometimes difficult to see that "letting go" is not the same as saying that something didn't hurt or wasn't a big deal. Explore the difference between acceptance and approval.

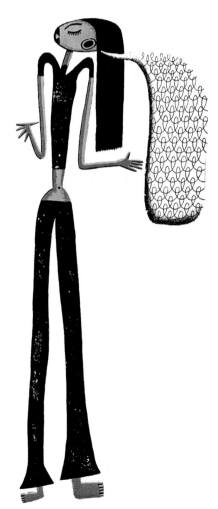

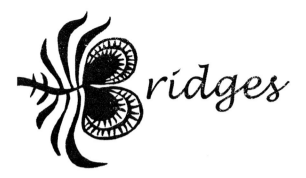

Bridges

ACTIVITY GOALS

Encourages problem-solving skills, allows the client to gain a greater perspective of their current struggles and life issues by defining a problem in words, shapes, texture and symbols. This exercise is a journey and an experience of moving from problem-focused thinking to solution-focused thinking. This progression instills hope and generates ideas for solutions.

NOTE: Clients suffering from terminal illness or other unchangeable life circumstance may need to focus on acceptance and letting go rather than a "solution."

IDEAS FOR VARIATION

- Ask the client to identify their support system and write about or draw them into the composition as well.

- Give the clients wire, clay or found objects and have them create the bridge and a figure of themselves in three-dimensional form. Ask the client take themselves on the journey figuratively and ask questions as they go such as: What do you see around you as you start out? What are you feeling?

- If the clients are in a recovery program, have them act the scene out as a journey activity. Ask the group to form two rows facing each other, creating a bridge. Ask one client to take a step towards the bridge, while their peers throw out a pertinent verbal obstacles such as "What are you going to do when someone calls you up to go drinking?" or "What are you going to do at a party when you see your old friends using?" Ask the client to respond. Each next step they take is dependent on if they successfully verbally overcome the last obstacle. If they don't have a response, you can ask others to offer positive and constructive suggestions. The success of this activity is based on how much trust you have established within the group.

OPTIONAL MATERIALS

Recycled materials to make sculptures (paper towel rolls, old CDs, cardboard boxes, egg cartons, twigs and twine, scrap fabric, aluminum cans, pliable wire, chicken wire, etc.), wire cutters, PVC glue; Clay, pottery tools, newspaper to protect surfaces

DISCUSSION POINTS

- The bridge is a metaphor for the client's sense of stability and security. Watch for how they create the bridge and where they place themselves on it. Have they begun the journey yet? Is it a long journey? What are the risks (what's under the bridge)? If they haven't started on the bridge yet, they may not yet know how they are going to achieve their goal.

- Notice how solid and stable the bridge is: how is it supported? Discuss how to strengthen the bridge to make their journey successful. Ask about their support system: what do they need to make it through? Have the client physically add more to their drawing or sculpture of the bridge to add more strength.

- **Q:** Where do you want to be? What will motivate you to get to where you want to go?

- **Q:** What will you bring with you in your backpack and why? Who will help you on your journey? How will they help?

- **Q:** What is it like to step off into the unknown? What role does trust play? How can you risk yet still feel safe? What makes the trip worth the risk?

- **Q:** How does fear keep us from taking the first step? Can we succeed without failure? How does success cause fear or additional pressure? Discuss fear of failure/success and the importance of perseverance.

- **Q:** Why are goals important? How do you make/keep goals? Is it okay if your goals are not realistic?

- **Q:** What new thoughts or actions should you adopt to make getting to your goal easier?

Glossary

ART THERAPY is a type of psychotherapy that uses imagination, art-making and creativity to increase emotional well-being. Art therapy combines traditional psycho-therapeutic theories and techniques with specialized knowledge about the psychological aspects of the creative process, especially the affective properties of different art materials. As a mental health profession, art therapy is employed in many different clinical settings with many different types of patients. Art therapy is present in non-clinical settings as well, such as in art studios and workshops that focus on creativity development.[7]

COGNITIVE-BEHAVIORAL THERAPY (CBT) has been demonstrated by many research studies to be the most effective approach for a variety of psychological problems. In CBT, the therapy relationship is collaborative and goal-oriented, and the focus is on thoughts, beliefs, assumptions and behaviors. The goal is for a person to develop more realistic and rational perspectives, and make healthier behavioral choices, as well as to feel relief from negative emotional states. Specific techniques, strategies and methods (cognitive restructuring, relaxation exercises, exposure work, assertiveness training, and more) are used to help people to improve their mood, relationships and work performance.[8]

EMOTIONAL INTELLIGENCE is the awareness, innate ability, sensitivity and potential to perceive, assess and positively manage one's emotions in a healthy and productive manner. There are believed to be four branches of mental ability:

1. Emotional identification, perception and expression
2. Emotional facilitation of thought
3. Emotional understanding and
4. Emotional management

FREE ASSOCIATION is the spontaneous, uncensored outpouring of whatever comes to mind without censorship or external direction, regardless of how apparently unimportant or potentially embarrassing.

---

7 http://www.psychology.org
8 http://www.cognitive-therapy-associates.com

A Therapist's Companion to Chill & Spill | page 38

GUIDED IMAGERY is the conscious use of the imagination to create positive images in order to bring about healthy changes in both body and mind. Many researchers believe that the mind responds not only to "reality", but to our construct of reality. The use of guided imagery can help reduce emotional arousal and can reframe circumstances through metaphor. It is helpful for clients who may need to "rehearse" in their imagination behaviors and/or feelings that they need to change. It has successfully been used to reduce stress, stimulate the immune system and relieve the effects of both physical and emotional illness.

MALADAPTIVE BEHAVIOR is behavior that is unsuitable, counterproductive or inappropriate to a given situation and interferes with or sabotages mental, academic, social or personal skills. An example is physical aggression or destructiveness to self, others, animals or property which requires protective intervention. Some maladaptive behavior can be an attempt to communicate stress or to avoid conflicts between body and psyche.

MANDALAS are usually a complex, circular design divided into four or eight parts. The word is Sanskrit for "healing circle", "essence" or "wholeness." Carl Jung used mandalas and described them as "vessels into which we project our psyche." In art therapy, they are often used as a centering activity to help reduce anxiety. They are found in nature, architecture, art and religious cultures throughout time (Hindu, Native American, Buddhist and Christian).

MULTI-FLOW MAPS are often used in schools to help the student analyze a cause and effect relationship. This helps them sequence what caused something to happen and notice the results of that event. Sometimes there are effects which, in turn, influence initial causes. This circular cause and effect relationship is called a feedback loop.

NARRATIVE THERAPY is a form of psychotherapy using narrative, which addresses the stories by which people live their lives. Narrative therapy seeks to be a respectful, non-blaming approach to counseling and accepts the client as the expert in their own life. Their stories contain meaning for the individual, based on his or her interpretation of events and experiences. The meaning in turn influences him or her, and can have significant effects and consequences for the person. Narrative therapy views the problem as separate from the person, and assumes that people

have many skills, abilities, beliefs and values that can help them to change their relationship with the problems in their lives. Through re-telling stories in therapy, one can find alternative ways of expressing the story, as in taking a different angle with a different thematic meaning, selecting events and experiences that are consistent with that thread, and developing the narrative accordingly. The therapist seeks to engage the person in richly describing and strengthening these new, preferred stories. The alternative stories that emerge during collaborative therapeutic conversations with the therapist help the person to break free from the influence of his or her problems (or problematic stories), and they are in line with how the person would like to be and live his or her life.[9]

REFLECTIVE DISTANCE is an art therapy term used to define the cognitive distance between the art experience and the individual's reflection of that experience; the ability to verbalize what they visually created; the ability to externalize feelings or traumatic events through non-direct means;[10] the ability of time to give perspective on a situation.

SURVIVAL VALUE is a concept in evolution linking survival of the fittest to natural selection. It describes healthy or unhealthy traits or behaviors that a person adopts with the positive intention of protecting and benefiting the person, allowing survival.

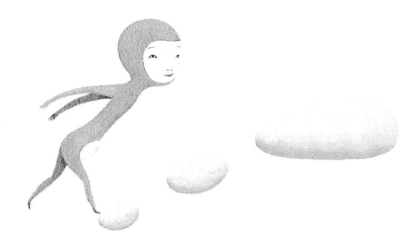

---

9 Ibid
10 Kagin, S. L. & Lusebrink, V. B. (1978). The expressive therapies continuum. The Arts in Psychotherapy, 5(4), 171-180

Stories from the Field

Crystal, MSW at the Renaissance Home For Youth in Alexandria, Louisiana was skeptical at first when she was first introduced to Chill & Spill. Some of the youth she works with are considered dangerous and are undergoing long term treatment and rehabilitation. "These teenagers are oftentimes afraid to trust and open up for fear of rejection, but I found that Chill & Spill helped them release these inner inhibitions. As a result, they've learned a lot about themselves and how to handle their feelings in a positive manner." One of the girls, "Laurie" was new and refused to talk to anyone. Crystal offered her the book and kept it safe from the others in her office. As Laurie worked through the book, the "Exclusive Interview" activity captured her imagination and she worked on it for a long time. "She had always been told that she was a trouble maker, that she was 'good for nothing.' This activity made her think about her strengths and talents, which made her realize that she did actually have something to offer. She now is outgoing and participates in activities. She even has a life goal now as a direct result of the book: she wants to be a pediatrician." Crystal also found it to be a useful tool for the teens to look back through the book to see what they wrote in the past and see how far they have come. "Chill & Spill has literally changed the way the teens respond to us and how we communicate with them."

Alisa Peterson, MSW, LICSW, a social worker at Hutch School in Seattle, Washington, gave a book to "Sally" during the weekly high school group for youth affected by cancer. Sally was a very private fifteen year-old whose mother was undergoing a stem cell transplant for leukemia. Sally finished "Inside of Me" during the group session and then volunteered to share her entry with the group. Sally shared that she was experiencing feelings of loss, fear, anger and hopelessness. Sally's sharing sparked a conversation amongst her peers that normalized her feelings and helped other students express themselves as well. The group committed to working on the entry throughout the week and sharing their work the next week. "As a group facilitator, it is exciting to see kids learn from each others' experiences and realize they aren't alone. This activity gave Sally and the other students a structure in which to write their thoughts and feelings. We use Chill & Spill every week in both the junior high and high school groups at Hutch School."

Heidi, a volunteer youth worker in Cleveland, Ohio, gave Chill & Spill to "Casey" to work on at home. Casey was a 16 year old student dealing with severe mental health issues. When Heidi sat down with her to discuss the book, Casey was in tears. She showed Heidi her drawings and it was immediately clear that she was in significant danger of hurting herself and others. She said it was too painful to discuss her drawings. Casey had used the book to draw her feelings instead of act on them. Heidi commented, "The book was a valuable tool in keeping Casey safe. I told her that she could use the book unconditionally, that she did not have to discuss her drawings with me," she continued, "I have since spoken with her case manager, and she is now taking the book with her to therapy sessions to help her deal with some of the more serious issues in her life." Heidi continues, "After seeing her drawings, I had a much better understanding her strengths and weaknesses. I was able to implement changes in the structure of her participation in our program which will make the experience safer and more productive for her."

Alicea Rieger, MEd ESA, works in a school setting in Bellevue, Washington. After working through Chill & Spill, "Chris" told her that she has been able to make new friends because she feels more confident in herself. Chris uses the book to express her feelings without being judged by others. Says Alicea, "I have found it valuable to have copies of Chill & Spill on hand. It is a great tool for students that need a safe outlet for their feelings. The book also gives students ideas on how to continue to help themselves in the future. I've received positive feedback from all the students I have given the book to. I plan on using the book in future groups as well as with individual students."

Linda Bordelon of The Orchard Foundation in Alexandria, Louisiana has given Chill & Spill to the school counselors and teachers she serves shortly after Hurricane Katrina hit. Says Linda, "The book allows kids to 'attack' their problems without intimidation or fear. Teachers and others who attended Art with Heart's training have taught others how to use the book with their students. It has made a difference in the way they perceive their plight and are more understanding that they are not hopeless. It has given them a better understanding and a resolve to deal with the current situation and work towards improving their outlook on life. They are coping better."

Diana, an 18 year old foster care teen and frequent Children's Hospital patient in Seattle, has used not one, but two, Chill & Spill journals. Having had both serious health problems and being in and out of the foster care system since she was eight, she has had her share of trauma, both physically and emotionally. Says Diana, "There are days when things are really bothering me and Chill & Spill gives me a good place to put everything down. It asks you to think about things and the changes you need to make in your life to make it better. I use it a lot to write about things that make me frustrated. Sometimes doctors do or say things that make me really mad, but instead of being mad, I can just write in Chill & Spill until I feel better. That way I don't lose friends because I'm grouchy." Recently, Diana saved up her disability paycheck to purchase books for other kids at Children's Hospital citing that the book had helped her so much that she wanted her friends still stuck in the hospital to benefit from it too.

DeAnn Yamamoto, MA, Director of Client Services at King County Sexual Assault Resource Center in Seattle, Washington wrote "Chris, our male educator who works with a middle school boy's group, took Chill & Spill with him for the first time. The day before, we had brainstormed about various scenarios that might happen and how he could facilitate the process. And, truth be known, he was preparing himself for the worst (in case the boys didn't like the book). Well, he came back AMAZED and DELIGHTED. The boys were thrilled from the moment they laid eyes on the book. They quickly took them out of the shrink-wrap and commented on every picture. Some of the kids started the first activity before Chris was even done handing them out. Chris had to shove the guys out the door because they wanted to stay and write, but if they did, they would have been late for class. He had to force them to shut the book and promise not to take it out in their next class!"

We want to hear from you!

Submit your story describing your experiences with this program, client successes and/or unique ways you use Chill & Spill for consideration in the next printing as well as on the website. Stories submitted are subject to editorial approval and editing for length and grammar.

Please submit your comments to chill@artwithheart.org or write to us at: Art with Heart, P.O. Box 94402, Seattle, WA 98124-6702.

About Art with Heart

Art with Heart is a nonprofit organization that empowers youth in crisis through therapeutic books and programs that foster self-expression. Traumatic situations can lead to emotional suffering. Art with Heart believes that by providing a creative outlet, youth will not just survive, but thrive.

www.artwithheart.org

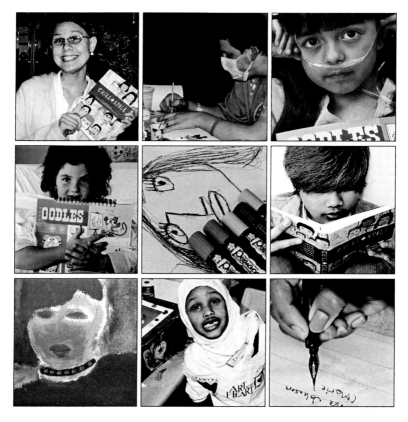

About the Authors

Jeanean Jacobs, MA, ATR-BC, CPC received her Master of Arts in Art Therapy at the University of Louisville in 1999. Currently, Jeanean serves as the Senior Director of Young Adult Services at the YMCA of Greater Seattle, helping young adults as they transition out of the foster care system. She is professionally certified as a Registered Art Therapist, National Board Certified Art Therapist, Professional Coach, Juvenile Sexual Offender Counselor and Life Space Crisis Intervention Counselor. She served on the board of directors of the Phoenix Institute in Kentucky and is a former board member of Art with Heart. She is a member of the American Art Therapy Association and lives in Seattle. She is passionate about helping young adults reach beyond difficult circumstances to create a life of their choosing.

Steffanie Lorig founded Art with Heart in 1996 while serving on the board of the Seattle chapter of the American Institute of Graphic Arts (AIGA). She is an award-winning author and graphic designer, as well as an illustrator and speaker. She received a Bachelor of Fine Art in Visual Communication from Northern Arizona University. After a successful career in the design world, she left to pursue Art with Heart full time and serves as their Executive Director. She is the visionary and author of **Oodles of Doodles for Your Noodle,** an activity book for seriously ill children, **Home Run Fun** an activity book for young Seattle Mariner fans. She is co-author of **Chill & Spill** through Art with Heart Press and she and her husband co-wrote a children's book called **Silly Baby** (Chronicle Books, 2008). She has served on the board of directors for the AIGA as well as the National Illustrator's Conference (ICON). Steffanie is a member of the Society for Arts in Health Care. Her creative work on behalf of children in crisis has been recognized by the national Make-A-Wish Foundation, the Lance Armstrong Foundation and the Starlight Starbright Foundation and she is the recipient of the Blair L. Sadler International Healing Arts award. Oodles of Doodles has helped over 20,000 hospitalized children since its first printing.

Ordering Information

1. CHILL & SPILL INDIVIDUAL ORDERS

Chill & Spill Journal: 14.2 oz, 5.5x8.5", 37 full color/70 blank pages

Chill & Spill individual cost.. $18.95 each

2. THERAPIST'S COMPANION

The Chill & Spill Therapist's Companion comes bundled with one PowerPoint CD to support group training

Therapist's Companion with Training CD .... $55 each
Therapist's Companion (no CD)..................................... $40 each

3. THERAPIST'S RESOURCE KIT

The kit covers nine Students and one Leader. It includes one Therapist's Companion book with Training Power-Point CD, nine Chill & Spill journals, ten C&S bookmarks and ten evaluation forms

Resource Kit.. $170 / kit

4. CHILL & SPILL BULK ORDERS

Bulk rate is applicable for orders **in increments of five** (40% discount). A case contains 32 books (48% discount).

Bulk rate (**in increments of 5 only**)................................ $11 / book

Case rate (32 books)... $315 / case

SHIPPING RATES

Box of 5 Chill & Spill .... $8 per box

Box of 20 Chill & Spill.. $17 per box

Case of 32 Chill & Spill .... $25 per box

Therapist's Companion (with or without Training CD) ...... $5 per set

Therapist's Resource Kit... $17 per kit

PLEASE NOTE: UPS Ground does not ship to P.O. boxes. Non-US orders may have additional customs fees, which we cannot calculate or foresee. **Canada, Alaska and Hawaii:** please add $10/box on all orders. **All orders are final.** See actual order form for complete listing of costs.

CONTACT

Art with Heart • P.O. Box 94402 • Seattle, WA 98124-6702
FAX: 206.277.7836 • PHONE: 206.362.4047
www.artwithheart.org • orders@artwithheart.org

ORDER ONLINE at **www.artwithheart.org/shop** or mail or fax completed form to:
Art with Heart, P.O. Box 94402, Seattle, WA 98124-6702 • FAX: 206.277.7836

ORDERED BY:

Name	
Organization	
Position/Title	
Address	
City/State/ZIP	
Phone	
E-mail	

SHIP TO (if different than ordered by)

Name			
Organization			
Address			
City/State/ZIP			
Phone		E-mail:	
How you heard about us:			

PAYMENT METHOD:

❏ Check/money order enclosed and made out to "Art with Heart" in US funds
❏ Visa ❏ MC   ❏ **PURCHASE ORDER #**

Card #			
Expiration		Security No.*	
Name on Card			

Security Number is the last 3 digits printed on the back of your credit card.

ORDERING INFO:

ITEM	BULK PRICE	TOTAL QTY	COST
Chill & Spill - individual rate	$18.95 each		
Chill & Spill Bulk Order	$11.00/book **in increments of 5**		
Chill & Spill Case Order	$315/case (32 books) *48% off retail*		
C&S Therapist's Companion	❏ $55 with CD ❏ $40 without		
C&S Resource Kit	$170 per kit (for 9 students, 1 leader)		
Canada, Alaska and Hawaii: please add $10/box on all orders		Subtotal	
Handling ($5 per order)			
Shipping (see chart on previous page)			
WA State Residents, Add 8.8% Sales Tax			
YOUR DONATION HELPS US HELP MORE KIDS			
		TOTAL	$

PLEASE TAKE A MOMENT TO FILL OUT THE FOLLOWING

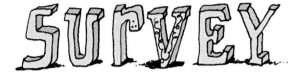

AND SEND IT TO US:

Art with Heart | P.O. Box 94402, Seattle, WA 98124-6702

email: info@artwithheart.org | www.artwithheart.org

phone: 206.362.4047 | fax: 206.277.7836

OR

SIMPLY FILL IT OUT ONLINE AT:

www.artwithheart.org/chillandspill

and click on the survey link!

Thanks!

Chill & Spill Therapist Companion Survey

 c/o: Art with Heart

P.O. Box 94402

Seattle, WA 98124-6702

PLACE STAMP HERE

Tape along bottom to seal